YOGA:
YOGA FOR BEGINNERS

10 Super Easy Poses
To Reduce Stress and Anxiety

Peter Cook

YOGA:
YOGA FOR BEGINNERS

10 Super Easy Poses
To Reduce Stress and Anxiety

Peter Cook

ERRORS

Please contact me if you find any errors.

My publisher and I have taken every effort to ensure the quality and correctness of this book. However, after going over the book draft time and again, we sometimes don't see the forest for the trees anymore.

If you notice any errors, I would really appreciate it if you could contact me directly before taking any other action. This allows me to quickly fix it.

Errors: errors@semsoli.com

REVIEWS

Reviews and feedback help improve this book and the author.

If you enjoy this book, I would greatly appreciate it if you were able to take a few moments to share your opinion and post a review online.

By The Same Author

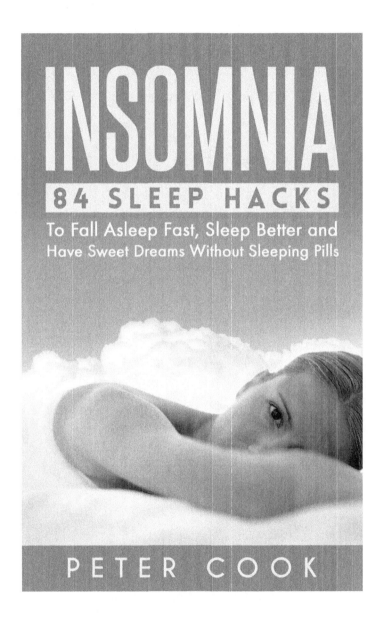

"Yoga doesn't bring you a sense of peace, health or well being. It's not like taking valium. Rather, it helps you quiet down your mind and body. So you can experience what your true nature is, which is to be peaceful until we disturb it."

Dr. Dean Ornish in the documentary 'Yoga Unveiled'

"To do is to be" - **Friedrich Nietzsche**
"To be is to do" - **Immanuel Kant**
"Do be do be do" - **Frank Sinatra**

Table Of Contents

Table Of Contents

It All Started on a Friday Afternoon…

It was an ordinary Friday summer afternoon and I was sitting behind my desk at the law firm I was working at. I was reviewing a contract for a client I had done a lot of work for over the last few months. I thought to myself: *"I can't believe I'm doing this work again. I'm so fed up with this!"* At that moment a headache started that would stay with me for more than one and a half years.

Hangovers aside, I never had headaches. So I didn't think much of it. I took it easy over the weekend, called in sick on Monday and Tuesday. On Wednesday I was behind my desk again. My boss was getting a bit worried: he was going on a holiday on Thursday and I had volunteered to supervise his files in his absence. So I did. Hey, this headache would go away soon, right? And it wasn't like I was having migraine attacks knocking me out on the floor. It felt more like a continuous pressure surrounding the back and side of my head, much like a laurel wreath.

By living on Paracetamol and Ibuprofen, I managed to get by during those three weeks. However, every evening I was completely exhausted. And I felt the same way on weekends. Clearly I wasn't healthy. So when my boss returned from his holiday, I cut my hours in half for a couple of weeks. This had no material effect. It was only then that I realized this wasn't just a regular headache: this was serious. To get healthy again, I had to stop working all together.

And so began a long period in search of recovery. At first I thought: perhaps it is a tumor, or cancer? Luckily, the results of the

11

hospital scans were negative. So what was it then? I quickly realized that Western medicine had no real answer and the only thing the doctors could offer me were painkillers. But that was just treating the symptoms, not the root!

I started going to the gym every day, doing intense workouts. Although the endorphins made me feel good afterwards, it didn't reduce my headaches. Interestingly, a psychologist even told me: *"You are doing the exact same thing with sports as you were doing at work! What you need is to learn to take things slowly."* So instead of going crazy in the gym, I started taking two-hour daily walks.

Over the course of these one and a half years I tried everything I could lay my hand one, like:

☐ Physiotherapy
☐ Exercise
☐ Volunteering as a dog walker at the local dog shelter
☐ Alexander technique
☐ Psychotherapy
☐ Stand up coaching courses
☐ Trigger point therapy
☐ Having the quality of my sleep researched in the hospital
☐ Craniosacral therapy
☐ Massage
☐ Changing my diet, including a ten-day vegetable juice fast
☐ Acupuncture

I even set aside the preconceptions I had about yoga. Like: *"Yoga is not masculine"*, *"I'm not flexible"* and *"I don't feel comfortable being in a class full of energy talking incense burning hippies while real men are lifting weights on the other side of the glass window in the same gym."*

12

Truth be told: yoga didn't do much for me at the time. I just went to a class a few times and was struggling a lot with the poses. I never got to the point where I could really focus my attention inwards, which I now know is the beauty of yoga. Nevertheless, it was my first introduction to yoga and it was enough to plant the seed for a much deeper practice later on in life.

After three and a half months, I went back to work again. Starting with four hours per week, the idea was to gradually build up the hours over the course of a couple of months. However, when I found that I wasn't even able to work more than twelve hours a week I realized it was no good. What can you really accomplish in this timeframe? And even in those twelve hours, I wasn't getting any serious work done. So I was back to square one and stopped working again. Depression was kicking in.

It wasn't until I did a ten day Vipassana meditation retreat that something really shifted for the first time. When I learned of these retreats, I immediately booked one. The start was horrible. At the airport I had to wait for five hours for a bus to take me to the retreat center in the middle of nowhere. I was very agitated: I hadn't slept well, my iPod had crashed, I obviously had a headache, children were crying, the speaker announced the same 'beware of pickpocketing' message every fifteen minutes. Aaaarrrggghh!

The retreat itself was intense: ten days of not talking, sitting in meditation for ten to eleven hours, in blocks of one to two hours. Everything was set up to facilitate bringing our focus inwards. No TV, phones or computers, no writing or reading. Men and women slept and ate in separate rooms, and every night there would be a lecture to help us deepen our meditation. Even though it was challenging, I totally loved it.

When I was back at that same airport to fly back home ten days later, I found that something magical had happened. The same kind of people were buzzing and hurrying around, I heard the same speaker announcements. Yet, instead of getting annoyed by the cries of a baby, now I felt empathy for its parents. Even the pickpocketing announcement didn't affect my state of mind. The pressure of the headache was still there, but at the same time I felt so calm, centered and…happy!

Realizing this, I started to cry. Tears just rolled out of my eyes. I hadn't shed a tear in years. So it didn't take long before that little voice in the back of my head started to comment: *"Stop crying, you're making a complete fool of yourself!"*. However, there was no stopping it. It lasted for almost two hours! *"This is crazy"*, I said to myself. I moved out of my chair and started walking back and forth through the terminal. If people were going to see my tears, at least it wouldn't be the same person sitting opposite of me for fifteen minutes straight! For the first time since the headaches began, I felt that I had tapped into something that could make me better.

After the retreat, my meditation practice kept me on my feet. When your life is shaken upside down like this, it is easy to get depressed. I had already started saving money to build a buffer for when I eventually would be fired. I seriously conceived that I may have to flip burgers at a McDonald's. Most days, I couldn't read for longer than thirty minutes per day, so any job position where I needed to use my intellect was out of the question. The uncertainty of my future - 'was I ever going to be free of headaches?' - was a new source of stress of its own.

The following example will give you an idea of how the headaches impacted my everyday life. I remember being at my parents' home for my dad's birthday. I was having a conversation with my mother. At one time, there were three different conversations going on between different family members. A healthy person would be able to automatically zoom in on the conversation he is involved in and zoom out of the others. I couldn't: I heard and followed every conversation at the same level at the same time. Consequently, my head felt like it was about to explode. I had to tell my mom to stop talking to me immediately, because I couldn't handle it. Ultimately - by trial and error and keeping an open mind - I did recover.

One of the most important lessons I learned was seeing how much the body and mind are connected. Where before I would just see my body as something that merely supports my head and should just do its job, I now started to have a much bigger appreciation for it.

I realized that the ultimate root of my headaches was not being on the right path. I missed a sense of purpose in my life: money brings comfort, but not true happiness. Now don't get me wrong: I don't think there is anything wrong with making money. However, in my personal life I have learned that I can no longer do a job that doesn't also satisfy certain inner values. Like touching another person's life in a positive way or feeling that the work I do makes a material difference in someone's life. As a lawyer, there had been so many moments where I asked myself: why am I doing this? Many times I wasn't able to answer this question in a satisfactory manner.

Here began my journey to pursue a life long dream to travel through Asia and ultimately finding yoga.

In yoga, many things that I had learned during my times of headaches came together. I learned how to quiet down the mind, how to listen and properly take care of my body, how the body and mind are interconnected. And I have learned the importance of a life with a sense of purpose. And these are not just intellectual teachings. These teachings are to be learned at an experiential level!

I started to develop my personal yoga practice. Also, I decided to anchor yoga in my life by doing an intense three months (550 hours) Yoga Teacher Training, followed by a two months (340 hours) Yoga Therapy Training. I started to teach. And now I want to share my experience and the knowledge I have gained over the years on a broader platform, in order to help anyone interested to improve their quality of life!

Nowadays, one of the most important causes of health problems is stress. Chances are that if you are reading this book, you are dealing with a certain level of stress in your life. If stress symptoms are not addressed adequately, they are likely to become chronic and ultimately lead to exhaustion. I know from personal experience that Western medicine often offers no adequate solution to stress. Yoga has been proven numerous times by Western science to reduce stress. It does so by taking a radically different approach. Dr. Dean Ornish said it wonderfully in the documentary 'Yoga Unveiled':

"Yoga doesn't bring you a sense of peace, health or well being. It's not like taking valium. Rather, it helps you quiet down your mind and body. So you can experience what your true nature is, which is to be peaceful until we disturb it."

I only wished I had learned about yoga earlier. When I suffered from my headaches, I often questioned the purpose of it all. What was I to learn from all of this? In hindsight, it is easy to say that this difficult experience taught me a lesson. Everyone loves a good 'falling down and getting back on your feet' story. However, when you are in the middle of that difficult experience and you have no way of knowing whether it is ever going to end, it is very difficult to have this perspective. So if you are in the middle of such an experience, I hope my story can be an inspiration to you.

If I hadn't gone through this journey, chances are that I would not have felt compelled to write this book.

It has now been about four years since my daily headaches stopped. I don't want you to experience what I have been through. Instead, I would like to help you reduce stress in your life by practicing yoga.
So let's get to it: are you ready?

Peter Cook

1. Introduction

Teacher: *"Ok class, I would now like to move into a tripod headstand. If you don't feel comfortable, there is no shame in just lying on your mat in child pose."*
Student: *"Lady, I got it."*
Teacher: *"Sir, if you just want to lay down in child's pose."*
Student: *"Shhpppppaaaaaa! Bring it, bring it!"*
Teacher: *"I don't want you to break your neck, so..."*
Student: *"What's up? My legs, that's what!"*
Teacher: *"We are doing a quiet headstand today."*
Student: *"I'm doing a handstand, mother**. I'm doing a handstand."*
Teacher: *"Ok, you know why don't we just release?"*
Student, while crashing down: *"Thank God!"*

Deleted scene from Forgetting Sarah Marshall (2008)

The Stress Test

Let's start with a little test. All I ask of you is to be honest. Not with me, but with yourself. Ready?

Ask yourself:

☐ Have you recently snapped (or even exploded) at someone over something small, like not doing the dishes?

☐ Are you feeling that you have too much on your plate and you don't know how to manage it?
☐ Do you often feel nervous or anxious?
☐ Do you worry a lot?
☐ Are you having trouble falling asleep?

If you answer one or more of these questions with yes, it is likely that you have been under too much stress for too long. Also, chances are that you are not taking adequate measures to reduce this stress.

I have good news for you though:

☐ You are not alone
☐ Reading this book and applying the yoga poses in it will help you significantly reduce your level of stress

You Are Not Alone

In November 2014, ComPsych® Corporation released a report with the results of a stress survey conducted among 1,880 American workers (https://goo.gl/SHqq4M). The survey showed that **64%** of employees report having **high levels of stress**, with extreme fatigue and feeling out of control.

In February 2015, the American Psychological Association released a report with the results of a stress survey conducted among 3,068 adults (https://goo.gl/8R3eOK). On average, Americans rated their stress level a 4.9 on a 10-point scale, where 1 is "little or no stress" and 10 is "a great deal of stress". This is higher than what Americans believe to be healthy — 3.7 on a 10-point scale. Some of the other findings of this survey include:

- **42%** of adults say they are **not doing enough** or are not sure
whether they are doing enough **to manage their stress.**
20% say
they are not engaging in an activity to help relieve or
manage their stress.
- The most commonly reported **sources of stress** include:
money
(64% report that this is a very or somewhat significant
source of stress), work (60%), the economy (49%), family
responsibilities
(47%) and personal health concerns (46%).
- The most commonly reported **symptoms of stress** include:
feeling irritable or angry (37%), feeling nervous or anxious
(35%), having a lack of interest or motivation (34%),
fatigue (32%), feeling overwhelmed (32%) and being
depressed or sad (32%).
- **41%** of adults who are married or living with a partner say
that they have **lost patience** or **yelled at their spouse or
partner** due to stress in the past month. And 18% of those
who are employed said they snapped or were short with a
coworker in the past month.

These are some shocking numbers!

Being under too much stress has a serious impact on every aspect
of your life. Being stressed out negatively influences your
relationships, your ability to enjoy things, your physical health,
your sex life, your performance and ultimately your experience of
life.

How This Book Will Help You Reduce Stress

In this book you will first learn what stress is. Also, you will learn that your perception of stress impacts the way you experience stress. I will then share with you ten simple yoga poses that can significantly help to reduce your stress if you practice them regularly.

Next, you will learn how yoga can reduce stress. Science has proven that practicing yoga reduces stress (https://goo.gl/ZOxb20). Yoga differentiates itself from other types of exercise in that it combines physical exercise with a mental awareness. The purpose of yoga is not to achieve a certain result. Instead, yoga teaches you to let go of any goal oriented mindset. Through yoga, you will learn how mind and body are in constant interaction with each other.

And finally, you will learn ten simple yoga poses that can significantly help reduce your stress when practiced regularly.

By performing these yoga poses, you will understand the power of yoga not just at an intellectual level, but at an experiential level. After all, are you ever going to know how a freshly brewed espresso tastes by only reading books about it?

Yoga Is For Women, Not For Real Men

In my experience, there are quite a few men who have all kinds of excuses why they won't do yoga. Although this book is written to help both men AND women, I want everyone to be on board before we get into the juicy stuff.

Some of the most common reasons men give when asked why they don't want to do yoga are:

1. Yoga is a feminine activity. The yoga studio is a women's space. I need to maintain my masculine image.
2. I am afraid of being perceived as a perve.
3. I am not flexible.

Let's address those:

1. Yoga is a Feminine Activity

Not true! Yoga is a practice that has roots that go back thousands of years. Yoga was actually developed by men and always practiced by men. Practically all the great classical teachers and writers of yoga have been men.

Only when yoga found its way to the U.S. in the 20th century, it somehow transformed into a form of exercise primarily practiced by women. Marketing can leave a big imprint on how we perceive things. When we read about yoga, we see an image of a fit and flexible woman practicing yoga on a magazine cover. And in that magazine you will probably find Lululemon's latest yoga pants advertisement. However, don't be fooled. Yoga is not simply gymnastics and is most definitely for both men and women.

Still not comfortable with the idea? Let it grow on you. It grew on me. You can practice the yoga poses in this book in the privacy of your own home. Don't let your pride stand in the way of this unique chance to significantly reduce your stress.

2. I am Afraid of Being Perceived as a Perve

This one is mentioned surprisingly often. Again, you can start practicing at home, where this will not be an issue. Also, if you go to a class, you will find that more and more men are doing yoga and most women actually appreciate men coming to a yoga class.

Finally, as you will quickly learn when you start practicing, yoga is very much an inner experience. Ten minutes into your practice, you will simply find yourself holding a pose, with your eyes closed and your focus inwards.

3. I am Not Flexible

"I'm too weak, so I can't lift weights."

Or what about this one: *"I'm too dirty, so I can't take a shower."*

See my point?

Let me add to this that the purpose of yoga is not to become more flexible, although this will be a side effect.

When I just started practicing yoga, I was very inflexible. When I bended forward, I could barely move my hands past my knees! After a lot of practice, I am now able to touch the floor with my fingertips. Yet, I sometimes see people come into the class who have never practiced yoga before and are nevertheless able to place their entire hands on the floor the first time they practice the forward bend.

At those times it is good to remember that yoga is not a competition. Leave your ego at the door. Yoga is a practice that connects the mind and the body by building an inner awareness. If you are under stress, this connection is often lost or weak. So yoga is <u>exactly</u> what you need, regardless of your flexibility!

What's Ahead?

Let's get to the meat and potatoes of this book. In the following chapters you will learn:

- ☐ What stress is
- ☐ How yoga can reduce stress
- ☐ Ten simple yoga poses that will significantly reduce your stress

I hope you are excited! But first, let's start off with a story.

2. A Walk Through The Jungle

Imagine it is the year 4,002 BC. There are no cities where you live. As a matter of fact, you have never even heard of the word city. Or anything else that we take for granted today: cars, phones, coffee, computers, croissants or airplanes. None of this stuff exists. Your life is basic and simple.

You are a hunter and live in a small tribe close to the woods. Your main purpose in life is to provide food for your loving family. The men of your tribe go out hunting a few times per week. Today is hunting day. This morning you and the other hunters left early.

There is just something to walking through the forest on an early morning: the trees are partly hidden by a mist. Everything smells fresh. The leaves are still covered with dewdrops. It feels a bit chilly this morning.

It doesn't take long before you find yourself separated from the other hunters. Not uncommon, nothing to worry about. You actually enjoy the stillness. As you move slowly through the trees, you are careful not to make any sound that might alarm the animals.

Then, all of sudden you hear a terrifying roar, look to your right and look straight into the eyes of a tiger!

Your response is automatic: **GO!! ALARM!!** You start running like Speedy Gonzales, your heart is beating like crazy, your senses are razor-sharp. Energy you didn't know you had keeps you running at a miraculous speed. Is the tiger still there? Keep running! You're breathing at a fast pace, your feet are bleeding by now, but you don't even feel it. All of sudden you see a big tree. You climb into it and move up quickly. Just in time; as you climb up, the tiger takes a jump. His open jaws just miss your feet!

You climb up further to a tree branch big enough to hold you and sit down on it. You lean back against the tree trunk, exhausted. Finally, you can relax a little. Your heart rate drops, the pace of your breath decreases.

After walking around the tree for a while, the tiger finally realizes he won't be eating this hunter for dinner tonight and moves back into the misty jungle...

3. What Is Stress?

"I am an old man and have known a great many troubles, but most of them never happened."

Mark Twain

Ok, you can take a few deeps breaths now. It was just a story!

What exactly happened to the hunter, standing in front of the tiger? You just imagined yourself being in his shoes. Although, come to think of it, he probably was barefooted. Anyway, the point I want to make is, do you think standing in front of a tiger is the right time to:

- ☐ think about that negative comment James made about you yesterday?
- ☐ cut your toe nails?
- ☐ take a nap?
- ☐ decide whether you want to order a pizza Salami or pizza Hawaii?

Of course not! The body of the hunter went into survival mode. When you sense danger - whether it's real or imagined - the body's defenses kick into high gear in a rapid, automatic process known as the "fight-or-flight" response. This is the first step of the stress response.

When you imagined yourself as the hunter, did you personally experience some of the physical symptoms, like an increased heart beat, shallower breath and tensed up muscles? Many people do. This clearly shows how mind and body are connected, something we will touch on in more detail later.

The Stress Response

The stress response is the body's way of protecting you. It helps you stay focused, energetic and alert. In emergency situations, stress can save your life. It will give you extra strength to defend yourself or spur you to slam on the brakes to avoid an accident.

The stress response helps you rise to meet challenges. For example, stress is what keeps you on your toes during a presentation at work. Or it sharpens your concentration when you're attempting the game-winning free throw.

But beyond a certain point, stress stops being helpful and starts causing major damage to your health, your mood, your productivity, your relationships and your quality of life.

For 99% of the species on this planet the stress-response lasts 3 minutes. After this, the threat is either over, or the animal is over and done with. However, we humans turn it on for a 30-year mortgage. That is not what the system evolved for. If you do this chronically, the stress response becomes more damaging than the stressor itself.

Two Types Of Regulation

The purpose of the stress response is to bring the body back to balance - the fancy term is: homeostasis - when a (perceived) stressor presents itself. How does it work?

There are two types of regulation involved in the stress response:

1. The nervous system
2. Hormones

1. The Nervous System

Simply put, there are two parts of the autonomic nervous system involved in the stress response:

- Sympathetic nervous system ("**SNS**")
- Parasympathetic nervous system ("**PNS**")

Often, the SNS is referred to as 'fight-or-flight', whereas the PNS is referred to as 'rest-and-digest'.

2. Hormones

The second type of regulation involved in the stress response are hormones. Hormones are chemical messengers that are blood borne, and as a result can affect events throughout your body.

The Stress Response In Action

When a stressor is perceived, the SNS is activated. The SNS sends a message to the adrenal glands on top of the kidneys, which then secrete epinephrine (also known as adrenaline). Another hormone that is secreted is cortisol.

This causes bodily changes:

- The heart rate and blood pressure go up

- The breath is more rapid

☐ Extra oxygen is sent to the brain, which increases alertness

☐ The senses, like sight and hearing, are more sharp

☐ Blood sugar (glucose) and fats are released from temporary storage sites, supplying energy to all parts of the body

These inbuilt functions are designed to help you fight or flee the tiger.

All these changes happen so quickly that you are not even aware of them. The wiring is so efficient that this process has started even before the brain's visual centers have had a chance to fully process what is happening. This is why you are able to run away from the tiger or jump out of the way of an oncoming car even before you think about what you are doing.

For the most part, the SNS and PNS work in opposition. This means that when the SNS is activated, the PNS is inhibited. The PNS mediates calm, vegetative functions like digestion, the secretion of insulin and the production of growth hormones.

Chronic Stress

In a healthy person, the sympathetic and parasympathetic nervous system are balanced. You need both, like you need a gas pedal and a brake to drive a car.

The stress response is elementary for your survival. Normally, no ill effects are experienced from the stress response. However, if your system keeps on stepping on that gas pedal there will be consequences. Your body is not designed to be in survival mode continuously. The stress response is intended for threats only.

Yet, many people are unable to find the brake. Chronic stress is fueled by mental activity, like continuously worrying about possible events. Imagine an engine that is idling too high for too long. This is when the stress response becomes more damaging than the stressor itself.

Chronic stress disrupts nearly every system in your body. If not addressed, it can eventually lead to:

☐ Burn-out

☐ High blood pressure

☐ Immune suppression

☐ Impaired digestion

☐ Diabetes

☐ Greater risk of chronic disease, even premature death

A tragic example of what can happen when you are under chronic stress is the story of Mita Diran, a young female copywriter for Young & Rubicam in Indonesia. In December 2013, she collapsed into a coma after working non-stop for three days. She died shortly afterwards. A colleague of her said she passed away due to a lethal combination of being overworked and excessive consumption of Krating Daeng (the Thai version of Red Bull energy drink). In her last tweet she said: "30 hours of working and still going strooong."

If you experience chronic stress symptoms, learn to listen to your body before it is too late.

4. Change Your Perception Of Stress

"Whether you think you can, or you think you can't: you are right."

Henry Ford

The Power of the Mind

In his book Unlimited Power, Anthony Robbins describes a case of a psychiatric patient with a split personality. One of her personalities was diabetic. Another personality was not. When she was in her non-diabetic personality, her blood sugars would be normal. However, when she flipped into her diabetic counterpart, her blood sugars rose. Also, all medical evidence demonstrated that she was diabetic. When her personality shifted back to her non-diabetic alter ego, her blood sugars normalized again…

This extraordinary example illustrates the power the mind can have over the body. In the prior chapter you learned that stress is the body's normal physical response to a threat. You also learned that when you don't know how to step on the brake, stress will cause a variety of symptoms ultimately leading to exhaustion.

In this chapter you will learn how you can use the power of your mind to reduce the stress symptoms you might experience. A lot of information in this chapter is inspired by the work of health psychologist and stress expert Kelly McGonigal. I highly recommend that, after reading this chapter, you also check out her books if you want to learn more about how your perception of stress impacts your experience of stress.

Your Perception of Stress Matters

How do you perceive stress? If you are like most people, you probably experience stress symptoms as negative and frustrating. Why can't these symptoms just go away?

If this thought pattern is familiar to you, you will benefit a lot from the lesson of this chapter:

You can reduce the negative experience of your stress symptoms by changing your <u>perception</u> of stress.

Sounds like some hippie airy-fairy BS? Think again. This statement is backed up by some serious scientific evidence.

The Belief That Stress is Bad For You Can Kill You

In a study conducted by the University of Wisconsin, researchers tracked almost 30,000 American adults for eight years (https:// goo.gl/OSsxtl). The researchers asked each person two questions:

1. how much stress have you experienced in the last year?
2. do you believe stress is harmful for your health?

Eight years later they checked the public records to find out who died. The results?

People that experienced:

36

- a lot of stress in the previous year and believed stress is harmful had a 43% increased risk of dying.
- a lot of stress in the previous year but did NOT view stress as harmful had the **lowest risk of dying** of anyone in the study. **Including people who experienced very little stress!**

Researchers estimated that over the eight years they were tracking deaths, 182,000 Americans died prematurely. Not from stress, but from the <u>belief</u> that stress is bad for you.

So that's one good reason to change your perception of stress: believing that stress is bad for you can kill you!

View Your Stress Response as Helpful

Imagine this: you are a salesman working for an advertising agency. The agency is struggling financially. Many companies have reduced their marketing budget and your advertisement agency is feeling the pain. This afternoon a meeting is planned with four representatives of Coca-Cola, the agency's biggest client. Recently, Coca-Cola has issued complaints about the quality of the advertisements created by you and your team. Your boss has expressed his concern that Coca-Cola might hire a competing advertising agency. If that were to happen, chances are that your agency will have to file for bankruptcy.

You have been chosen to be the star of the show this afternoon. In the last few weeks, you have been preparing yourself for the moment of truth. It's all on your shoulders. Little does your boss know that you absolutely despise giving presentations. Moreover, you once had a panic attack in college while giving a presentation. Now, each time when you are put in front of a group the fear of shutting down is there, ready to choke you.

Only five more minutes until the start of the meeting. Your heart starts to pound, the pace of your breath increases, your skin gets warm and sweaty, your hands start to shake. You hate this feeling, why can't you just feel relaxed?

Normally we view these physical changes as anxiety, or signs that we aren't coping well with the pressure. But think about this for a second: what if instead you viewed these changes as signs that your body is getting energized, preparing you to meet the challenge ahead?

This question was researched in a study conducted by Harvard university (https://goo.gl/Nh3lf5). Students participating in the study had to go through a social stress test. Each student was tasked with giving a five-minute speech on their personal weaknesses to a panel of expert evaluators. To add to the pressure, the students had to stand in front of a camera and bright lights. To make matters even worse, the evaluators had been trained to give the students discouraging non-verbal feedback. The second part of the study was a math test, in which the evaluators had been trained to harass the student during it. You can imagine the stress symptoms the students were experiencing!

The interesting part of this study is that a portion of the participating students had been told to rethink their stress response as helpful. The results of the study were remarkable. Students who learned to see stress as helpful were less stressed out, less anxious and more confident. The most fascinating result of this study however is that their **physical stress response also changed!**

During a typical stress response, the heart rate goes up and the blood vessels constrict. This is why sometimes chronic stress is related to cardiovascular disease. The blood vessels of the students who viewed their stress as helpful did not constrict, but stayed relaxed. Their heart was still pounding, but this was a much healthier cardiovascular profile. Over a lifetime of stressful experiences, this one biological change could be the difference between a stress induced heart attack at age fifty and living well into your nineties.

So how you think about stress matters!

Care About Others to Build Stress Resilience

The last scientific study that I want to share with you shows that caring about others creates stress resilience (https://goo.gl/YtKUYT). How does this work?

In a study conducted by the University of Buffalo, 1,000 adult Americans were asked the following two questions:

1. How much stress have you experienced in the last year?
2. How much time have you spent helping out friends/neighbors/people in your community?

As in the first study, the researchers checked the public records to find out who had died five years on.

The study results showed that every major stressful life experience increased an adult's risk of death by 30%. However, this was not true for those that also spent a significant amount of time helping loved ones and neighbors. In those cases, there was a **0% increase in risk of death**.

So you actively build your stress resilience by caring about others!

How Can You Apply This in Your Daily Life?

Let's summarize the findings of these three studies:

1. The belief that stress is bad for you can kill you
2. Viewing your stress response as helpful reduces your stress symptoms
3. Caring about others builds stress resilience

Harmful effects of stress on your health are **not inevitable**. How you **think** and how you **act** can transform your experience of stress.

But how can you apply this in your daily life?

Next time when you are under stress, smile and think:

"Look, this is my body preparing me. It is giving me energy. It helps me stand up to this challenge."

When you view stress in this way, your body believes you and your stress response becomes healthier. And if you want to build your stress resilience even further, make sure you spend time loving and caring about others.

5. Yoga Reduces Stress

"I did a sequence of poses this morning that only ten people on the planet can do, ending with the corpse pose. Do you know what I've done with yoga? I beat it. It's time to move on, to something more ultimate."

From the action movie Faster (2010)

So far, you have learned that stress is the body's normal physical response to a threat. Also, you have learned that changing your perception of stress has a big impact on how you experience stress symptoms.

In the next chapter you will learn ten yoga poses that will significantly reduce your stress symptoms when practiced on a regular basis. But first you will learn how yoga can reduce stress.

Isn't Yoga Just Another Form of Exercise?

Numerous scientific studies have shown that practicing yoga reduces stress. For example, one study in which students performed ten weeks of classroom-based yoga showed that the levels of the stress hormone cortisol had decreased significantly and that the students' behavior improved. You can find more examples of scientific studies later on in this chapter.

But doesn't any exercise reduce stress? Wouldn't playing a game of basketball or lifting weights at the gym equally reduce stress?

41

Let me start by saying that I highly recommend you practice any form of sport. It will get you in shape, get your blood pumping and make you feel good.

Yoga however is unique in that it combines physical exercise with a mental awareness. In practically all other exercises there is a goal to be achieved or a challenge to be met. Like winning a game or building muscle strength. In yoga however, there is no such goal. Yoga merely uses physical exercise as a tool to create a balanced mind.

There is scientific evidence that yoga can have a stronger effect on a person's sense of well-being than other forms of exercise. For example, one study showed that regular yoga practice increases brain GABA levels and improves mood and anxiety more than other metabolically matched exercises such as walking.

Taking a look at the origins of yoga may show why yoga has a much more profound stress reducing effect than regular exercise. If you are not interested in - or feel uncomfortable with - the spiritual aspects of yoga, don't worry: the ten yoga poses you will learn in the next chapter do not require any spiritual aspiration. However, to understand how yoga techniques are different from regular exercises, you need to know why these techniques were created in the first place.

The Origins of Yoga

Yoga is a practice with roots going back thousands of years. The reason it works so well for stress reduction is because its primary focus is building awareness, not fitness. Yoga was designed as a path to realize the true nature of one's self; or in other terms, enlightenment. The word yoga means 'union' which refers to union of body, mind and soul; and of oneself with the origin of creation.

The purpose of traditional yoga is beautifully illustrated in the work 'Three aspects of the absolute' by the artist Bulaki.

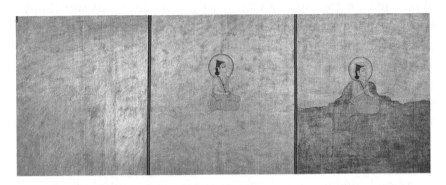

'Three aspects of the absolute' (1823), Bulaki

The panel on the right shows a yogi sitting on the ground, meditating with a golden sky around him. The golden sky represents the infinite, the ground the material finite world. In the second panel, he has drifted away from the ground, expanding his consciousness. In the last panel, only a luminous sea of gold remains: the yogi has entirely disappeared into enlightened self-realization.

The practice originally focused primarily on the mind, not physical transformation as we customarily find in our western yoga studios.

Over time, Tantra yoga was developed, which accepted that this world is a manifestation of the ultimate reality. We have to accept our condition here, but we have to understand it differently, in a transfigured way. This practically means seeing the divine source in everything around you. Think of how a young girl explores the world around her. She can be completely captivated by the small wonders of this world, like the beautiful colors of a flower, or a beetle racing through the grass. We can all practice this in our daily lives.

Tantra yoga introduced a new relationship to the physical body. Where the ascetic paths saw the body and its desires as something that needed to be transcended, tantra yoga teaches that there is only one supreme reality, and it includes our bodies and our world. Consciousness and matter are not separate, but two ends of one undivided spectrum, like two poles of a single magnet. Hence, the body was seen as a temple of the divine which needed to be kept fit to prepare it for spiritual realization.

This led to the creation of Hatha yoga, which is a vast collection of exercises including asanas (poses), pranayama (control of prana, the subtle energetic streams in the breath), bandhas (body locks) and mudras (hand gestures). By practicing these exercises, in combination with the other eight limbs described by Patanjali in his Yoga Sutras, such as concentration of the mind and meditation, the practitioner aimed to acquire self-knowledge and ultimately realize his or her true self.

However, it was not just a matter of doing the practice, and then expecting to automatically achieve self-realization. Ultimately, self-realization was a gift bestowed upon the practitioner by grace. Therefore, persistence in practice was no guarantee of enlightenment, and practice best went hand in hand with detachment to the outcome.

All physical yoga styles we see in Western yoga classes today use poses that originate from Hatha - and thus Tantra - yoga. Styles like Ashtanga, Vinyasa Flow, Power yoga or Yin yoga, to name only a few. A good analogy would be to compare Tantra yoga to water and the many different styles to drinks like coke, orange juice or coffee. Each drink has a different flavor, but its core ingredient is water.

How Does Yoga Reduce Stress?

In an interview with Forbes magazine, Paula R. Pullen (PhD, Research Instructor at the Morehouse School of Medicine) describes yoga as follows:

"Yoga balances the body, the hormonal system, and the stress response. People tend to think of yoga as being all about flexibility – it's not. It's about rebalancing and healing the body." (https:// goo.gl/htvwNt)

The healing benefits of yoga have been shown by numerous scientific studies. In addition to the studies (https://goo.gl/3Ao0pq) mentioned earlier in this chapter, scientific studies have shown that yoga:

☐ reduces levels of the stress hormone cortisol. Consequently, the immune function is boosted.
☐ boosts levels of feel-good brain chemicals like GABA, serotonin, and dopamine. These chemicals are responsible for feelings of relaxation and contentedness, anxiety control and the way the brain processes rewards.
☐ stimulates the parasympathetic nervous system, which calms us down and restores balance after a major stressor is over.

Let me give you an example. In a study conducted by Thomas Jefferson Medical College in Philadelphia and the Yoga Research Society (https://goo.gl/54MNcg), sixteen healthy subjects who were new to yoga participated in a fifty-minute yoga class every day for seven days. Prior to the start of their first class, they were instructed to sit quietly, reading and writing, for fifty minutes. The subjects' cortisol levels didn't change appreciably during the sitting period. They showed just the normal decrease that usually takes place in the late morning. But when the researchers measured the cortisol levels before and after the yoga class, they discovered a significant decrease after the class.

The findings of this study suggest that practicing yoga - even for the very first time! - can normalize cortisol levels that are either too high or too low, according to Vijayendra Pratap, Ph.D. (president of the Yoga Research Society in Philadelphia).

In a Yoga Journal article (https://goo.gl/hLTkmT) on de-stressing with yoga, Jennifer Johnston (yoga director and research clinician at the Mind Body Medical Institute in Boston) adds to this:

"The deep breathing we do in yoga elicits something called 'the relaxation response,' which invokes the restorative functions of the body. Yogic practices also help to reduce muscle tension and deactivate the stress response."

Chronic stress is fueled by mental activity, such as continuously worrying about possible events. Yoga changes the mind patterns, by practicing awareness of our thoughts and detachment. On the mat yoga offers momentarily relief. Ultimately it is transformative because it helps you to have better future reactions.

The Ego is Not Your Amigo

In our Western society we are flooded with images of super flexible or strong people performing incredible yoga poses. Yoga may seem like just another form of exercise in which people compete to become the best, strongest, or most flexible.

Although it can be beautiful to see a person perform a challenging yoga pose perfectly, yoga was not created to transform a person into an acrobat. Its purpose was to help the practitioner realize his inner nature by bringing balance to the mind and body.
Awareness is the most important feature of yoga. The body and mind are constantly interacting with each other. If you practice yoga, this will no longer be only an intellectual concept, but something you will experience within. As the famous yoga teacher Swami Sivananda of Rishikesh said: *"an ounce of practice is worth more than a ton of theory."*

Many busy people are often very much 'in their head' so to speak and less in touch with their body. When I was a lawyer I basically saw my body as a means to get me to meetings. I would get angry if I got sick. As if my body was letting me down, whereas in reality I wasn't respecting my body. By focusing your attention on the breath or a body part, you restore the connection between mind and body. When you calm the body down with awareness, you also calm the mind.

When practicing the forward bend pose, for example, it is completely irrelevant whether you can place your hands flat on the floor or are only able to extend to the level of your knees. What matters is your state of mind.

Remember, unlike other forms of exercise, yoga is not about pushing far beyond your physical limitations, but about transforming the mind. If you compare yourself to those around you that are more flexible, this will negate the purpose of the exercise. Realizing that "your ego is not your amigo" as a friend once told me, you'll be well on your way to reducing the harmful stresses of life and making space for a calmer happier version of yourself to arise.

In the next chapter you will learn how you can start to build your own practice with ten simple yoga poses that will reduce your stress symptoms if practiced regularly. I hope you are excited!

6. Ten Super Easy Yoga Poses To Reduce Stress and Anxiety

Introduction

Let's practice some yoga together! I hope you are excited. The following ten yoga poses will significantly reduce the stress symptoms in your body. The poses are:

1. Breath awareness: Being aware of how you breathe is important in every yoga pose.

2. Surya Namaskara (Sun Salutations): This is a sequence of moving poses, which is really good to warm up the body.

3. Garudasana (Eagle Pose): This pose helps ward off stress by improving concentration and balance.

4. Jivabalasana (Life Force Pose): This is a static pose that can be challenging to hold for longer periods of time. It is a good pose to practice detachment and equanimity.

5. Marjariasana and Bitilasana (Cat / Cow Pose): This is a moving pose that brings great relief to tension in the back.

6. Balasana (Child's Pose): This an easy relaxation pose that feels very safe.

7. Viparita Karana (Legs Up The Wall): This pose is one of the best poses for stress reduction, because it is easy to perform and can be held for a long time.

8. Nadi Shodana Pranayama: This exercise deeply relaxes the body and mind.

9. Shavasana (Corpse Pose): This the ultimate relaxation pose.

10. Meditation: in meditation, you simply sit quiet and observe your mind.

Don't be put off by the use of the Sanskrit names. The reason that the Sanskrit names are included here is to avoid confusion. Often you will find that the Sanskrit name of a pose is translated in different ways.

For example: ex-pro wrestler Diamond Dallas Page is now a yoga teacher. For his DDP Yoga, he has rebranded the names of many poses. Balasana for example, which is commonly translated as 'Child's pose', is called 'Safety Zone' in DDP Yoga. By using the Sanskrit name in this audiobook, you will always be able to find relevant information about the correct asana.

For all yoga poses, I strongly advise you to keep your eyes closed (with the exception of the third yoga pose, Garudasana, or the Eagle Pose). This helps calm the mind by blocking out visual distractions. Also, keeping your eyes closed helps you to internalize your awareness, feel your body more and observe your thoughts.

Nevertheless, in case closed eyes produce internal discomfort, anxiety or any other unpleasant sensation, feel free to keep the eyes open, or better: half open, while attention still dwells inside the body.

How Should I Practice a Yoga Pose?

Later on in this chapter, you will find ten simple yoga poses that will reduce your stress symptoms if practiced regularly. Most of these poses are asanas. But what is the right way of practicing an asana?

Patanjali, author of the classical text Yoga Sutras, tells us that an asana should be **stable** and **comfortable** (Sutra II.46).

When you move into an asana, focus your attention on how your body feels. You can push a little till the limit of comfort. However, don't force anything. Accept the limitations of your body. Over time, you will become more flexible if you relax into the asana.

Now scan your body. Often we tense up moving into an asana. Don't hold onto this tension, but release it. Breathe deeply and slowly. Tell yourself to relax. When you are comfortable in the asana, it is important that you remain aware. Remember that yoga is not so much a physical exercise, but much more a practice in awareness. If you find yourself thinking about what you are going to have for dinner, or about that annoying colleague of yours who is always complaining about everything, bring your attention back to your body.

You might experience shaking of certain body parts while holding asanas for longer amounts of time. This is normal: don't give in immediately when the shaking starts. However, if you find that your body starts trembling uncontrollably, or your breath becomes irregular, you are pushing it too far. Come out of the pose. Patanjali warns: shaking of the body and irregular breathing cause distractions which agitate the mind and consciousness (Sutra I.31). The purpose of yoga is the opposite: the stopping of the fluctuations of the mind (Sutra I.2).

Practicing yoga on a regular basis will restore and deepen the connection between your mind and body. Also, your body will adapt. What seems as a difficult asana in the beginning will become easier to perform over time. Finally, by keeping a regular practice you will find that gradually you will be able to expand the stillness you experience on the mat into your life off the yoga mat.

1. Breath Awareness

Breathing deeply is key to relaxing the body and calming the mind.
A person under stress tends to have shallower breath than a relaxed
person. Therefore, during your yoga practice always be aware of
how you are breathing. For example, when you move into a
challenging pose you might find yourself tensing up. When you
become aware of this, consciously relax your tensed body parts
and breathe deeply into your abdominal area. This will make it
easier to go deeper into the pose.

How To Practice

Make sure you sit comfortably. You can sit on a cushion on your
yoga mat or on a chair, both are perfectly fine. Straighten your
back. Close your eyes. Place your left hand on your heart and your
right hand on your belly. Breathe naturally.

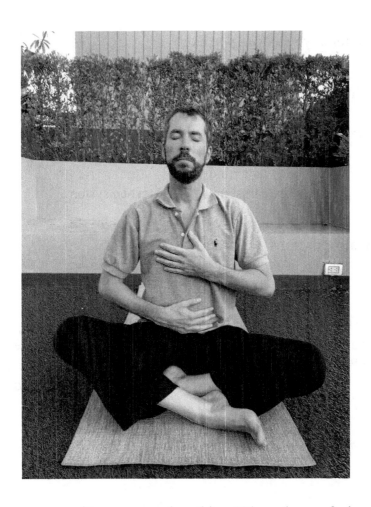

Become aware of how you are breathing. Where do you feel your breath? Is your belly moving when you inhale, or do you feel the expansion more in your chest area? Is the breath fast or slow? Whatever you observe, try not to judge or change it. Accept that this is how you are breathing in this moment.

Now bring your awareness to your belly and breathe deeply into it. Feel how your belly expands when you exhale, and moves back in when you inhale. Make your exhalations longer than your inhalations, as this relaxes your body.

Repeat for as you long as you like.

Benefits

The practice of the Breath Awareness:

- ☐ relaxes body and mind
- ☐ activates the parasympathetic nervous system

Contraindications

- ☐ None

Proper breathing is important in each of the other nine yoga poses. For example, when you move into a challenging pose like the Eagle Pose, your muscles might tense up. When you become aware of this, breathe deeply, and consciously relax your tensed body parts. This will make it easier to go deeper into the pose.

2. Surya Namaskara (Sun Salutations)

Sun Salutations are a common sequence of asanas. There are many variations. Well known examples are Sun Salutations A and B, which are for instance practiced in Ashtanga and also many Vinyasa Flow classes.

Here we will practice Sun Salutations A. In many yoga classes you will hear the Sanskrit names of the yoga poses. Therefore, I have included them here too. Again, if the names seem complicated, just disregard them. There is no exam at the end of this book!

Practice a minimum of six rounds. To deepen the experience, keep your eyes closed. You can keep them (half) open if you feel like you're losing your balance.

How To Practice

2.1 Tadasana (Mountain Pose)

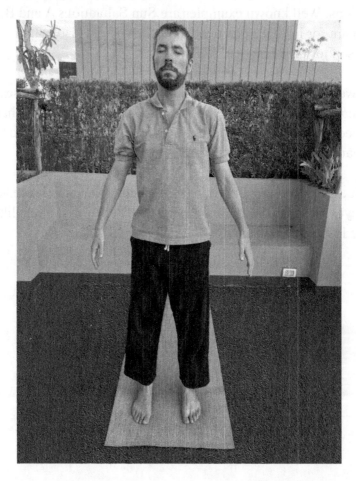

Stand with your feet parallel, close but not touching. Distribute your weight evenly over both feet. Hang your arms beside your torso. Establish a slow, steady rhythm for your breath. Find your center.

2.2 Urdhva Hastasana (Upward Salute)

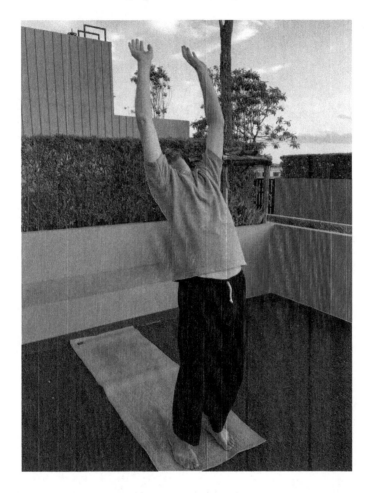

Stretch your arms out to the side and overhead. Bend the head, arms and upper trunk slightly backward, arching the spine.

2.3 Uttanasana (Standing Forward Bend)

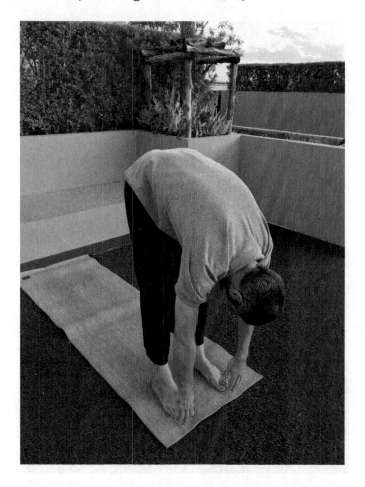

Hollow out your belly and fold forward. Keep your legs firmly engaged. Don't force your forward bend. If you can't reach the floor, so be it. Remember that yoga is not a flexibility contest. It is much more important to build body awareness and practice detachment. The ego is not your amigo!

2.4 Ardha Uttanasana (Half Standing Forward Bend)

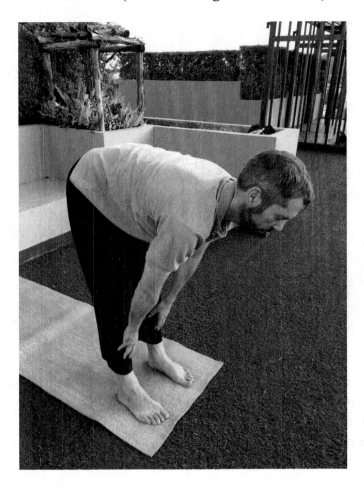

Inhale and lengthen your spine forward. Extend your spine. Your fingertips can stay on the floor or on your shins.

2.5 Chaturanga Dandasana (Four-Limbed Staff Pose)

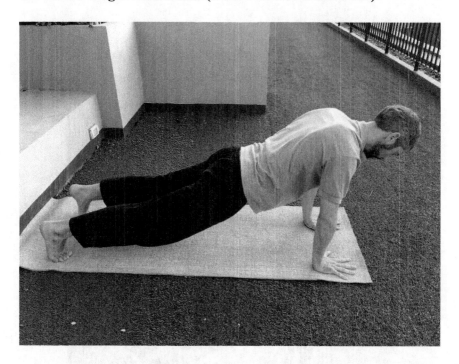

The next position resembles a plank. Step your feet back behind you. Your hands should be flat on the floor at shoulder-distance. You can spread your fingers to balance yourself and release pressure. Your feet should be at hip distance. Lengthen through your spine.

Now lower yourself. Keep your legs straight. Push back into your heels. If this is too hard, you can bring your knees to the floor.

2.6 Urdhva Mukha Svanasana (Upward-Facing Dog)

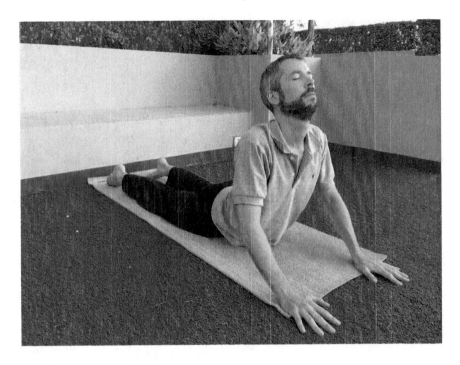

Place the top of your feet flat on the floor. Draw your chest forward. Pull your shoulders back and open your collar-bones. Engage your legs. Relax the muscles in your buttocks, pelvic floor and upper legs.

2.7 Adho Mukha Svanasana (Downward-Facing Dog)

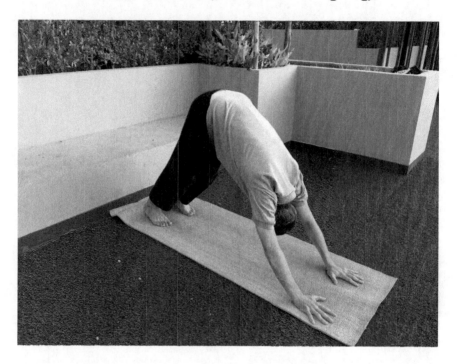

Roll over your toes. Ground down through your hands and feet as you lengthen your spine. Gaze backwards between your toes. If you find that your weight is resting on your hands, your weight is too far forward and you need to push back a little. Remain here for at least five breaths.

2.8 Ardha Uttanasana (Half Standing Forward Bend)

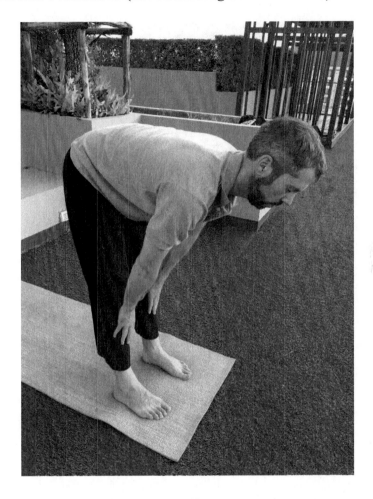

Bend your knees and look between your hands. Step or lightly hop your feet between your hands. Move back into Half Standing Forward Bend (no. 2.4 above).

2.9 Uttanasana (Standing Forward Bend)

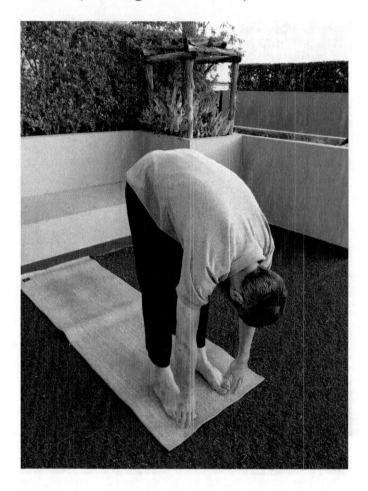

Bend forward into the Standing Forward Bend (no. 2.3 above).
Surrender to the fold.

2.10 Urdhva Hastasana (Upward Salute)

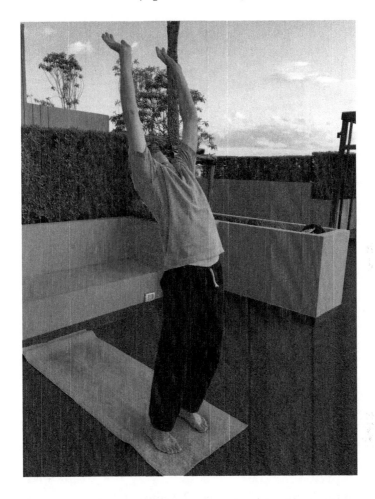

Reach your arms out wide to your sides and come up. Move into
Upward Salute (no. 2.2 above).

2.11 Tadasana (Mountain Pose)

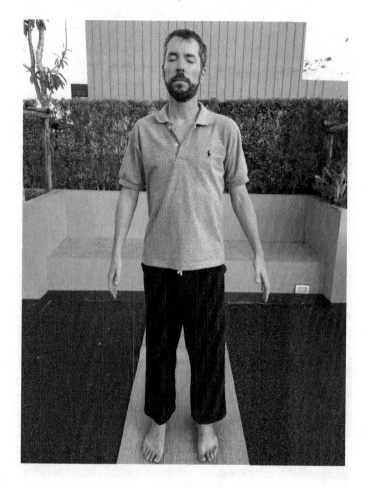

Return to the Mountain Pose (no. 2.1 above).

Don't immediately move into the next round of Sun Salutations. Instead, remain with your eyes closed and take a couple of breaths. Awareness is the most important aspect of your yoga practice. Feel the effect of this round before you move into the next one.

Benefits

The practice of the Sun Salutations:

- strengthens the back
- thoroughly ventilates the lungs and oxygenates the blood
- improves muscle flexibility
- stimulates and balances all the systems of the body, including the autonomic nervous system

Contraindications

- Hernia
- Severe renal disorders
- Pregnant women should not practice after first three months
- If you have high blood pressure or a heart disease, consult with your physician before practicing

3. Garudasana (Eagle Pose)

This is an active and empowering pose that can help ward off stress by improving concentration and balance. It also opens up the shoulders, upper back and hips.

How To Practice

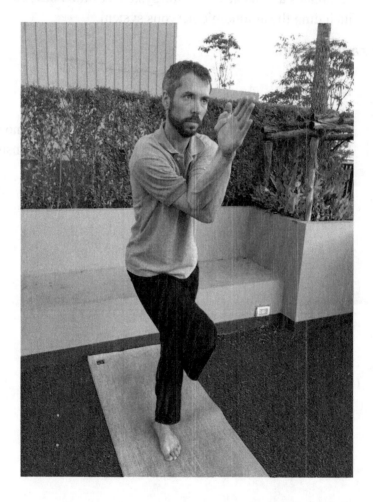

In this pose, it is necessary to keep your eyes open in order to maintain your balance.

It can be a bit complicated to get into this position. Take a good look at the photos to make sure you get it right. Start in a standing position. Bend both knees. Lift your right leg and wrap it around your left leg over your left thigh, hooking your right foot behind the left calf as deeply as possible. Balance on the left foot.

Now do a similar movement with your arms. Raise your left arm in front of your body to shoulder height, with the palm facing inward. Twist your right arm underneath it and wrap it around your left arm. Raise your right hand to clasp your left hand thumb with the index and middle fingers of your right hand. Then push the arms forward as much as possible, stretch the left palm, and straighten your spine to a vertical position.

Choose a point in front of you to focus on, just above the level of your eyes. This will make it easier to keep your balance. It is best to choose a point placed at a distance which roughly equals the height of your body. Make sure your hands are not blocking your view.

To come out of the pose slowly unwind your arms and then your legs. Come back to a neutral position.

Now repeat the asana on the opposite side, standing on your right leg.

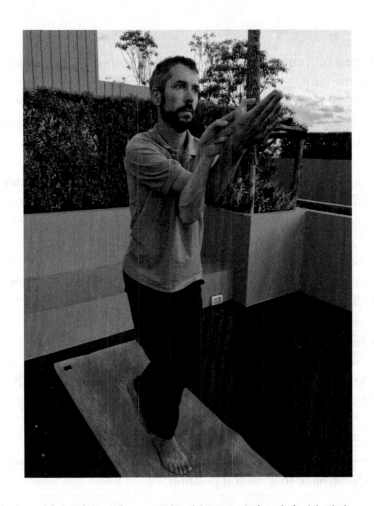

Variation: if the foot of your raised leg can't hook behind the calf of your standing leg, press the foot to the side of your leg or place the toes of the raised foot on the ground for balance.

Benefits

The practice of Garudasana:

☐ improves concentration
☐ improves balance

- strengthens and opens up the shoulders, upper back and hips
- strengthens and stretches the ankles and calves

Contraindications

- Knee injury: practice the variation

4. Jivabalasana (Life Force Pose)

This pose is physically demanding when held for a few minutes or longer. Because of its challenging nature, it is a good pose to practice detachment and equanimity.

How To Practice

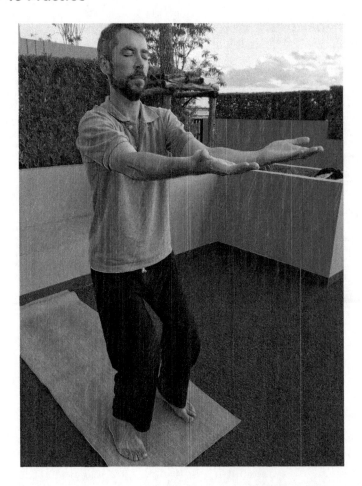

Stand with your feet parallel, shoulder-width apart. Bend your knees, as if you want to sit on a chair. Lift your arms and stretch them out in front of you, to shoulder height. Your palms are facing up. Relax your shoulders and fingers. Your spine should be vertical. Make sure your head is in line with your spine and neck. Relax all unnecessary muscles. Close your eyes.

When your arms or legs start to shake, don't stop performing the pose. Instead, bring your attention to the painful body part. Breathe deeply and try to relax the tension in your muscles.

Hold Jivabalasana for at least two minutes.

Benefits

The practice of Jivabalasana:

- deepens the mind and body connection
- strengthens joints, arms, legs, shoulders and chest
- helps with shaking arms and legs
- removes lethargy
- improves overall energy of your body
- improves blood circulation and stimulates the heart
- increases inner strength and determination
- trains the autonomic nervous system

Contraindications

- None

5. Marjariasana/Bitilasan (Cat/ Cow Pose)

This combination of two yoga poses is a gentle exercise that can bring great relief to any tension in the back.

How To Practice

Start on your hands and knees in a table-top position. Place your hands directly under your shoulders, your knees directly under the hips. Your head is in a natural position in line with the spine. Close your eyes.

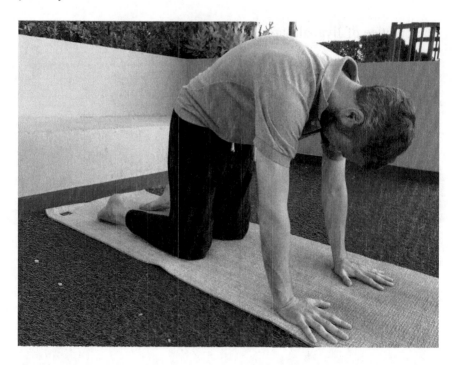

Marjariasana: On the exhalation, round your spine upwards and tuck your chin towards the chest. Contract your abdomen to expel as much air as possible from your lungs. Drop the pelvis towards the floor.

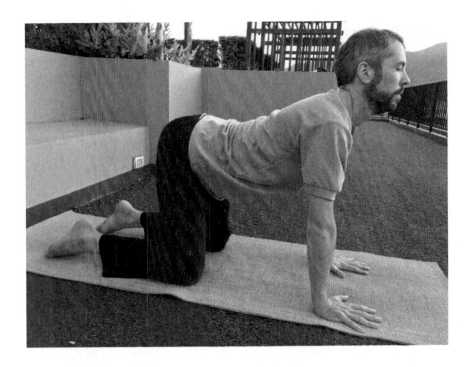

Bitilasana: On the inhalation, raise your head and pelvis upward and arch your spine in the opposite direction. Move your belly towards the floor. Relax your abdomen as you inhale.

Repeat at least ten times.

Benefits

The combined practice of Marjariasana and Bitilasana:

- [ ] stretches the back torso and neck
- [ ] releases tension in the spine
- [ ] is good training for the full abdominal breathing used in pranayama
- [ ] provides a gentle massage to the internal organs in the abdominal and pelvic regions

Contraindications

☐ With a neck injury, keep the head in line with the torso.

6. Balasana (Child's Pose)

Balasana is a resting pose. This pose feels very safe, because it resembles the fetal position in a mother's womb.

How To Practice

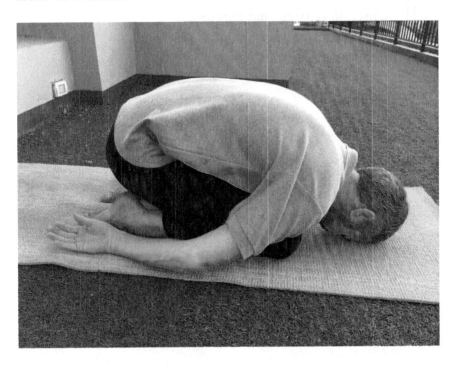

Sit in a kneeling pose with your knees together. Lean forward, resting your forehead on the floor. If possible, keep your buttocks in touch with your heels. Lay your hands on the floor, alongside your torso, with the palms up. Release the fronts of your shoulders toward the floor.

Hold for as long as you like.

Benefits

The practice of Balasana:

☐ vitalizes depleted nerves and glands
☐ has an overall positive effect on the entire body
☐ calms the brain
☐ helps relieve stress and fatigue
☐ relieves back and neck pain
☐ helps in case of insomnia

Contraindications

☐ Diarrhea
☐ Pregnancy
☐ Knee injury: avoid Balasana unless you have the supervision of an experienced teacher

7. Viparita Karana (Legs Up The Wall)

This is one of the best yoga poses for stress reduction. It is easy to perform and can be held for a very long time, even by people who have never practiced yoga before.

How To Practice

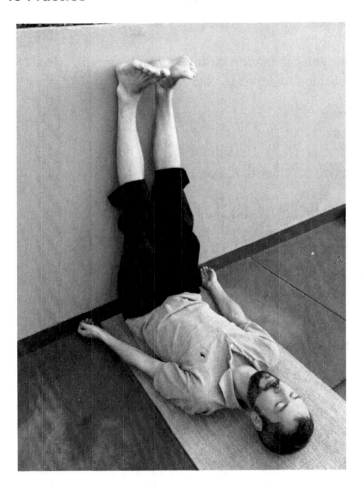

Place your yoga mat perpendicular to the wall. Lay on your right side, with your buttocks touching the wall. Turn yourself on your back. When you are lying on your back, stretch your legs and make sure they are completely against the wall. Place your arms next to your body and relax.

Try to not let your thoughts drift. Instead, focus your awareness on feeling your body. You could try to scan your body (see description of yoga exercise 9. Shavasana). Alternatively, focus your attention on the breath going in and out. When you find your mind has drifted off, don't get angry. Simply bring your attention back to the breath.

Variation: you can place a cushion under your hips. Also, you can place a cushion underneath your head.

Benefits

The practice of Viparita Karana:

- ☐ helps renew blood and lymph drainage back into the heart area
- ☐ relieves anxiety and depression
- ☐ reduces fatigue
- ☐ alleviates insomnia

Contraindications

- ☐ None

8. Nadi Shodana Pranayama (Alternate Nostril Breathing)

Nadi Shodana is a breathing technique in which you alternate breathing through your nostrils. This breathing technique deeply relaxes body and mind.

How To Practice

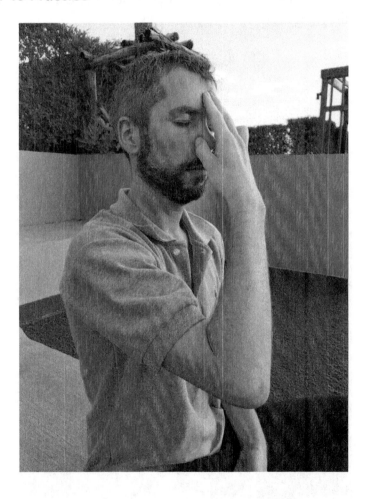

Sit in a comfortable position. It is perfectly okay to sit in a chair. Throughout this practice, use what you have learned in the Breath Awareness to breathe deeply into your abdominal area. Close your eyes.

- ☐ Block the right nostril with the thumb of your right hand and inhale through the left nostril.
- ☐ Next, release the thumb and now block the left nostril with the ring and little finger of your right hand. Exhale through the right nostril.

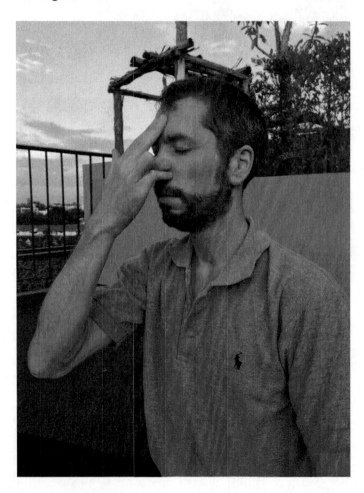

- ☐ Keep the left nostril blocked, inhale through the right.
- ☐ Block the right nostril and exhale through the left.

This is one round. Make sure you finish your last round with an exhalation through the left nostril.

Practice for at least five minutes.

Benefits

The practice of Nadi Shodana:

- ☐ calms down the nervous system
- ☐ increases concentration and focus
- ☐ regulates insomnia and hormonal imbalance
- ☐ balances your entire being
- ☐ balances the two brain hemispheres

Contraindications

- ☐ The practice of this pranayama can have a strong purifying effect, especially if you are a smoker. If you start to feel dizzy, stop the exercise.
- ☐ Make sure that you are not sitting close to any sharp edges, like the corner of a dining table. In the unlikely event that you faint, you don't want to hit your head on sharp edges!

9. Shavasana (Corpse Pose)

Shavasana seems like an easy pose to perform. You just lie on your back, right? However, it is considered the hardest yoga pose to perform correctly. Why is that?

The purpose of Shavasana is to consciously relax the body without falling asleep, letting go of everything. Many people are not able to do this. And when they are able to let go, they tend to lose consciousness and fall asleep.

What's so special about this pose? Isn't Shavasana just the same as relaxing on the couch? Science says no! Already in the mid 1970s, a study by Dr. Chandra Patel on the effect of Shavasana was published in The Lancet. Patel randomized 40 hypertensive persons to either:

☐ practice Shavasana, or
☐ relax lying on a couch

for half an hour, three times per week, for three months. The results showed that the subjects who had practiced Shavasana had a much higher drop in their blood pressure than the subjects who had just relaxed on a couch.

The difference between Shavasana and lying on the couch consists in what you are doing with your mind. Shavasana is a conscious relaxation where you use the mind to feel and relax the body.

How To Practice

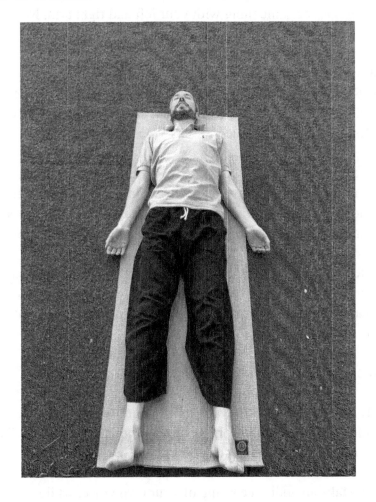

Lie on your back. If it makes you feel more comfortable, put a
pillow under your head and cover your body with a blanket. Spread
your legs slightly apart. Place your arms next to your body, let your
hands rest on the floor. More than in any other pose, it is important
to close your eyes.

Feel your body becoming heavy. Breathe deeply. When you are
ready, start scanning your entire body. Start with your left leg,
beginning at your toes and ending at the top. Feel how your left leg

is relaxed, while your right leg is not yet relaxed. Now relax your right leg. Do the same thing with your left and right arm. Now feel how all your limbs are relaxed.

Continue by relaxing the muscles in your buttocks and your pelvic floor. Relax your abdominal muscles. Continue with the muscles in your chest area. Relax your lower back, slowly moving your way up. Now relax your shoulders. Relax your throat and neck.

Relax all the muscles in your face. Now relax specific muscles in your face. Relax your jaw and cheeks. Relax your tongue. Relax your nose and ears. Relax your eyeballs and eyebrows. Relax your forehead, your temples. Relax the muscles on top of your head.

Now feel how your whole body is relaxed. Don't end Shavasana. Stay with the feeling of relaxation, with full awareness. Try to find that state where you are as relaxed as you can possibly be, without falling asleep.

Practice for at least ten minutes.

Tip 1: Before you start Shavasana, lift your arms and legs up. Contract all your muscles for five to ten seconds. Now let go. This way you are able to relax even deeper.

Tip 2: Make an audio recording of your own voice, while instructing the body scan. This way, you can follow your own instructions during Shavasana and go deeper into the relaxation.

Benefits

The practice of Shavasana:

☐ relaxes body and mind and restores their connection

- □ helps reduce high blood pressure
- □ relieves anxiety and depression
- □ reduces chronic fatigue
- □ alleviates sleeping disorders

Contraindications

- □ None

10. Meditation

There are many forms of meditation practices. What most practices have in common is a:

☐ narrowing of focus that shuts out the external world
☐ stilling of the body

In meditation, you will truly learn the nature of the mind. A common metaphor for the mind is a drunken monkey jumping around. To make matters worse, he also just got stung by a scorpion! Does that sound familiar?

Meditating after a busy day at work can be really challenging. Therefore, I recommend to meditate after an asana and pranayama practice. This releases tension and balances the body. Then meditation becomes much more powerful.

How To Practice

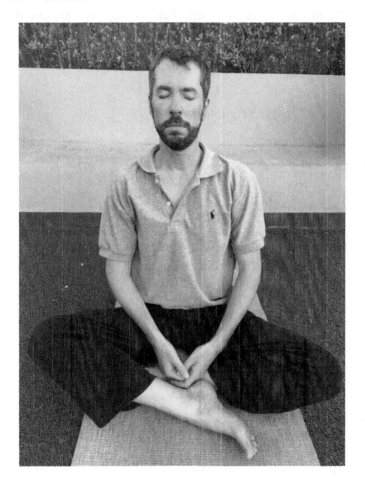

Sit in a comfortable position. It is perfectly okay to sit in a chair. Close your eyes.

Become aware of your pose. Make any necessary adjustments, so you can sit still during your meditation. Once you feel comfortable take a couple of deep breaths. Exhale deeply a few times. Now let the breath flow naturally. Observe your breath coming in and going out. If it helps you, count to ten and back.

After you have done this, remain still and observe whatever is coming up in your mind. The idea here is that you observe without identification and judgment. You will inevitably loose your focus, which might take some time to realize. When you do, just observe this and try again.

Practice for at least ten minutes.

Benefits

The practice of meditation:

- [ ] calms the mind, improves ability to concentrate
- [ ] train non-reactivity to thought activity
- [ ] lowers blood pressure
- [ ] boosts immune system
- [ ] has an anti-inflammatory effect

Contraindications

- [ ] None

7. Amplify The Effect: Combine The Yoga Poses!

The true power of these ten yoga poses lies in practicing them in the given order. This will really amplify the effect! Try to practice the sequence at least two times per week.

Sit in a space where you will not be disturbed. Turn off your phone. Begin with setting an intention to be fully present during this practice.

Then start with the Breath Awareness. Many people with chronic stress tend to breathe fast and shallow, primarily in their chest area. In a relaxed body, the breath is deep and slow. It is important to keep the breath deep and slow during your entire yoga practice. Alternatively, you can even choose to start in Shavasana, tense all the muscles for five seconds and then let go. Then move into a sitting position and perform the Breath Awareness. Practice the Breath Awareness for at least two minutes.

Next up are six rounds of Sun Salutations. The practice of Sun Salutations warms up and releases tension in the body. The Sun Salutations activate the sympathetic nervous system. Since a number of the other asanas activate the parasympathetic nervous system, the Sun Salutations give balance. After finishing six rounds, stand still for a minute and perceive the effect of the Sun Salutations.

Now start with the asana portion of the practice. Perform Garudasana (Eagle Pose), Jivabalasana (Life Force Pose), Marjariasana/Bitilasana (Cat / Cow Pose), Balasana (Child's Pose) and Viparita Karana (Legs Up The Wall). Hold every asana for at least one minute. The effects will be stronger if you hold the poses for two minutes or more. After each exercise, take a minute to feel the effect of this asana on your body and mind.

Come up to a seated position. Make sure you sit comfortably. You can sit in a chair. However, when you do, don't lean backwards: make sure your spine is straight. When you are ready, start the alternate nostril breathing exercise Nadi Shodana. This pranayama is especially powerful when preceded by an asana practice. Practice for ten minutes. When you finish, take a minute to feel the effect of Nadi Shodana.

Now lie down and relax in Shavasana (Corpse Pose). Close your eyes. Relax every muscle. Feel your body becoming heavy, sinking into the floor. Now perform the body scan. It would be great to use an audio recording of a body scan. Practice for at least ten minutes: don't rush Shavasana!

When you have finished Shavasana, come back to a seated position and end the practice with Meditation. Remain in the same seated position. Simply observe anything that comes up without judgment. Remember that drunken monkey stung by a scorpion? Meditate for ten minutes.

When you finish, remain seated for a while. Observe the effect, not only of this meditation, but of your whole practice. Compare how you feel now to how you felt before the practice, is there a difference? Is there a change in the level of stress you are experiencing right now? Finish by expressing gratitude for your practice. Try to maintain this awareness and apply it in your everyday life. As you build your yoga practice, you will find that this will become easier and easier. Consequently, your levels of stress will also reduce.

8. But I Don't Have Time For All That...

The ten yoga poses are especially powerful when practiced in the given sequence. But, what if you don't have the time to practice all of them?

First ask yourself, do you REALLY not have the time, or are you giving other things a higher priority? And are these things more important than freeing yourself of stress symptoms and being in good health? Remember, yoga is not a magic pill. It will only work for you if you commit to the practice. But if you do, yoga will significantly reduce your stress.

If after asking this question you still find yourself short on time, here's what you can do. In order to reap the benefits of the ten yoga poses, it is very important that you are calm and present when you perform them. Therefore, instead of rushing through all ten poses, it is better to remove a few asanas. Keep following the same sequence.

If you are really short on time and can't do more than one exercise, practice Shavasana. This is the most important yoga exercise in the list. You will get much better results from only practicing Shavasana well for ten minutes, than doing three other asanas in the same amount of time.

9. Bonus 1: Five-Minute Exercise Routine You Can Do Behind Your Desk

When you are working behind your desk all day, you're sitting in the same position for a long time. With this five-minute exercise routine, you will give your upper body a nice stretch and also improve your posture.

For all exercises, sit up straight, with your feet firmly placed on the floor.

1. Arm Stretch. Stretch your arms above your head and intertwine your fingers with the palms facing upward. Stretch your palms up to the ceiling and hold for a few seconds. Let go of the stretch, but keep your arms above your head. Then stretch your palms up to the ceiling again. Perform ten times.

2. Hand Clenching. Hold both arms straight in front of the body at shoulder level. Open the hands, with the palms facing each other, and stretch the fingers as wide apart as possible. Next, close the fingers to make a tight fist with the thumbs inside. Now open your hands again. Perform ten times.

3. Shoulder Rotation. Lift your shoulders up and then let them drop. This will relax them. Now slowly rotate the shoulders backwards, in a circular motion. Perform ten times. Next, rotate the shoulders forwards. Also perform ten times.

4. Spinal Twist. Exhale and slowly rotate around your axis to the left side of your chair, starting from the lower back and slowly moving up along the spine. Don't start with your head. Wait with rotating your head until you've fully rotated your spine. Place your left arm on the back of the chair, and your right arm on the left armrest. Be gentle, don't force the stretch. Keep breathing while you hold the spinal twist for a few seconds. When you come out of the twist, start from the top and work your way down the spine. Now perform the spinal twist on the opposite side. Perform five times on each side.

5. Side stretch. Place your hands in your sides. Now raise and stretch your left arm and move it over your head, with your upper body bending to right. This gives a nice stretch to the left side of your upper body. Hold for a few seconds. Place your left hand back into your side. Now perform the side stretch on the opposite direction. Perform ten times.

It will take no more than five minutes to perform this exercise routine and you will feel so much better after doing them!

10. Bonus 2: Did You Know These Things Also Release Stress?

Did you know that the following things are also known to release stress?

- ☐ Singing
- ☐ Massage
- ☐ Playing with kittens
- ☐ Forgiveness, compassion
- ☐ Orgasm
- ☐ Laughter
- ☐ And…Dark chocolate! (well, according to a study by chocolate producer Nestlé that is…)

11. Final Words – Now It Is Up To You

Congratulations! You have made it to the end of this book.

Let's recap what you have learned by reading this book:

- ☐ stress is the body's normal physical response to a threat. Only when you don't know how to step on the brake, stress becomes chronic and causes a variety of symptoms ultimately leading to exhaustion.
- ☐ your perception of stress matters. Don't perceive stress as something that is bad for you. Instead, view your stress response as helpful, and build your stress resilience by caring about others.
- ☐ yoga reduce stress. Unlike most other forms of exercise, the purpose of yoga is not to achieve a certain result. Instead, yoga teaches you to let go of any goal oriented mindset. Through yoga, you will learn how mind and body are in constant interaction with each other.
- ☐ ten yoga poses that will significantly reduce your stress symptoms when practiced regularly.

Now it is up to you. Roll out your yoga mat (or buy one if you don't have one yet) and start practicing the ten yoga poses you have learned. Keep in mind that yoga is not a magic pill. Yoga is much better than that. Yoga reduces your stress by letting you experience what your true nature is, which is to be peaceful.

Try to bring the awareness you practice, and the experience on your yoga mat, into your daily life. Often, we are not fully experiencing the present moment. Sitting in the car, you might be thinking about the groceries you need to pick up. In the grocery store, your thoughts are drifting towards the meeting you need to prepare for. In the meeting, you realize that you have forgotten to buy pasta for tonight's dinner...

This continuous mental activity is the fuel for chronic stress.

By practicing yoga on the mat, you learn to become aware of what is happening right now in your body and mind. The present moment holds stillness and joy, regardless of external circumstances. There can be no chronic stress in a person who is consistently fully present.

So even when you find yourself short on time, you can practice yoga by becoming aware each and every moment. Whether you are in a meeting or in the grocery store, observe how you feel and what comes up in your mind.

The ten yoga poses in this book are relatively easy to perform. There are many more asanas and other yoga techniques that are more challenging. However, when you are living a very stressful life, it is important to first learn how to relax your body. The ten yoga poses you have learned in this book will help you do this. Start with building body and mind awareness by practicing them. Once you feel that the practice starts having effect, there is nothing holding you back from exploring all the other beautiful techniques that yoga has to offer.

Remember, you don't have to be a victim of your stress symptoms. Reducing back stress is simply a matter of combining small steps. Take it one step at a time. When you fall down, get up again. Success consists of getting up just one more time than you fall. Just make sure you keep on walking. And take the first step today!

12. What's Next?

So where to go from here?

Join me in the complimentary video course **Yoga For Beginners: 10 Super Easy Poses to Reduce Stress And Anxiety**! It's hosted on Udemy, the *biggest* online learning platform.

You can access it at by going through this shortened link: **https://goo.gl/bTi4Cs**. It will take you directly to the course page on Udemy.

This course normally goes for $200. But as a reader of this book, I'm offering it to you at a **95% discount**.

You can get in for **just $10.99!**

Here's the link again: **https://goo.gl/bTi4Cs**

If you're asked to fill in a coupon code, use this: **YOGASTRESS**

By taking this video course, you will be able to deepen your understanding of the concepts you learned in this book:

- Ten Simple And Easy Yoga Exercises to Eliminate Stress and Anxiety
- What Stress Is
- What Yoga is
- How Doing Yoga Can Reduce Stress
- Why Yoga Differs From Other Types of Exercise in Reducing Stress and Anxiety
- And Much More Valuable Content!

We will go over each yoga exercise in detail. You will learn exactly how to perform them, and how they can help you reduce stress and anxiety.

The exercises you will learn in this course are easy. You do not need to be flexible and you do not need to have any prior yoga experience: this course is suitable for all levels!

The focus is on learning how to relax. People that experience a lot of stress are often not able to fully relax their body anymore. Even when they think they are relaxing, they still hold on to tension.

The purpose of the yoga poses in this course is to restore the connection between your body and your mind. If you practice these poses on a **regular** basis, I **promise** you that you will start feeling the beneficial effects **immediately**!

So…ARE YOU READY TO TAKE ACTION?

Then head on over to **https://goo.gl/bTi4Cs,** join me and let's continue our learning time together!

13. BONUS CHAPTER: How Much Sleep Do We Need?

Below, you will find a free bonus chapter from my popular book '***Insomnia***: *84 Sleep Hacks To Fall Asleep Fast, Sleep Better and Have Sweet Dreams Without Sleeping Pills*'.

Enjoy!

It is my way of saying thanks for

- ☐ reading this book, and
- ☐ starting your yoga practice. You rock!

Let's get started, shall we?

***

"One of the Georges - I forget which - once said that a certain number of hours' sleep each night - I cannot recall at the moment how many - made a man something which for the time being has slipped my memory."

P.G. Wodehouse, Something Fresh

<u>***Key Takeaway***</u>: *Most people need around 7-8 hours of sleep. Short sleepers can be categorized in two types: natural and habitual short sleepers. Natural short sleepers are rare, but due to a gene*

mutation they reap the benefits of a full night of sleep in nearly half the time. Habitual short sleepers on the other hand have trained themselves to sleep less. However, they take a risk, as they are not immune to the long-term risks of keeping themselves awake.

Introduction

In his book 'Think Like a Billionaire', Donald Trump wrote: *"Don't sleep any more than you have to, I usually sleep about four hours per night."* And when he was at an event in Springfield, Illinois campaigning for the 2016 elections, he said: *"You know, I'm not a big sleeper. I like three hours, four hours, I toss, I turn, I beep-de-beep, I want to find out what's going on."*

And Trump is not the only one with this sleep habit. Other people that have been reported to sleep as little as four hours a night are:

- **Thomas Edison,** producer of the first commercially viable light bulb, and inventor of the phonograph
- **Martha Stewart,** business woman, founder of Living Omnimedia and award-winning television show host, entrepreneur and bestselling author
- **Indra Nooyi,** Chairperson and Chief Executive Officer of PepsiCo

And in his book 'The 4 Hour Body', Tim Ferriss writes about sleeping less by using what is called the Uberman Sleep Schedule. This is a polyphasic sleep schedule consisting entirely of 20-minute naps, for a total of just three hours in six portions distributed equally throughout the day.

The implicit message of the likes of Donald Trump and Martha Stewart is that success can only be achieved by giving up hours of sleep. So is everyone who sleeps more than that just lazy?

The simple answer is: No.

***

The Average Adult Needs Seven Or More Hours Of Sleep Per Night

There may be a small percentage of people that are naturally short sleepers. But most people need around eight hours of sleep. In fact, in a June 2015 Sleep Journal publication, the American Academy of Sleep Medicine (AASM) and the Sleep Research Society both recommend at least seven or more hours of sleep per night for adults aged 18 to 60 years, to avoid the health risks of chronic inadequate sleep (goo.gl/yFR7lw).

When commenting on this publication, Dr. Nathaniel F. Watson of AASM said:

"Sleep is critical to health, along with a healthy diet and regular exercise. Our Consensus Panel found that sleeping six or fewer hours per night is inadequate to sustain health and safety in adults, and agreed that seven or more hours of sleep per night is recommended for all healthy adults."

***

But What About Short Sleepers?

Short sleepers can be categorized in two types:

105

- natural short sleepers
- habitual short sleepers

***

Natural Short Sleepers

Natural short sleepers are rare, but they do exist. They carry a mutation of the so-called DEC2 gene. The first scientist to publish about this was Ying-Hui Fu, a geneticist at the University of California at San Francisco. In a 2009 Science article (goo.gl/p8gi1P), she reports finding a mother-daughter pair who could both get away with only six hours of sleep. Without any ill effects. After examining their genes and comparing it to other test subjects, Fu found that both mother and daughter had the same mutation of the DEC2 gene.

So basically, natural short sleepers reap the benefits of a full night of sleep in nearly half the time.

***

Habitual Short Sleepers

Habitual short sleepers on the other hand are those that have trained themselves to sleep less. There are many different ways of training yourself to sleep less than seven to eight hours per night. From just getting out of bed every morning at 5 a.m., to following the Uberman Sleep Schedule. It takes some time for the body to develop and adapt to the new habit of short-term sleep. For example, when following the Uberman Sleep Schedule, people report feeling like a zombie for the first three to four weeks. But after a while they will be able to conquer the short-term effects of being sleep deprived, like lack of focus, bad mood, et cetera.

However, habitual short sleepers take a risk. Although they may attain short-term benefits, such as increased productivity, they are in danger of suffering long-term health consequences. They do not have the DEC2 gene mutation and are therefore not immune to the long-term risks of keeping themselves awake. The brain needs a full seven to eight hours of sleep every night in order to flush out chemicals it doesn't need, and to recharge. By not allowing this process to complete, habitual short sleepers put themselves at increased risk for a number of diseases, such as Alzheimer.

***

Get Enough Sleep

So are Donald Trump or Martha Stewart natural or habitual short sleepers? Who knows...

But for most of us it is safe to assume that we are not natural short sleepers. And while there are definitely short-term benefits to establishing a short sleep habit, you may put your long-term health at risk.

And to give you a final push, here is what Arianna Huffington wrote about getting enough sleep in her book 'Thrive':

"We think, mistakenly, that success is the result of the amount of time we put in at work, instead of the quality of time we put in. Sleep, or how little of it we need, has become a symbol of our prowess. We make a fetish of not getting enough sleep, and we boast about how little sleep we get. I once had dinner with a man who bragged to me that he'd gotten only four hours of sleep the

night before. I resisted the temptation to tell him that the dinner would have been a lot more interesting if he had gotten five."

So listen to your body, and make sure to get seven or more hours of sleep per night.

***

This is the end of this bonus chapter.

Want to continue reading?

Then get your copy of "Insomnia" at your favorite bookstore!

Did You Like This Book?

If you enjoyed this book, I would like to ask you for a favor. Would you be kind enough to share your thoughts and post a review of this book? Just a few sentences would already be really helpful.

Your voice is important for this book to reach as many people as possible.

The more reviews this book gets, the more people will be able to find it and reduce their stress through yoga.

***

IF YOU DID NOT LIKE THIS BOOK, THEN PLEASE TELL ME! You can email me at **feedback@semsoli.com**, to share with me what you did not like.

Perhaps I can change it.

A book does not have to be stagnant, in today's world. With feedback from readers like yourself, I can improve the book. So, you can impact the quality of this book, and I welcome your feedback. Help make this book better for everyone!

Thank you again for reading this book and good luck with applying everything you have learned!

I'm rooting for you…

By The Same Author

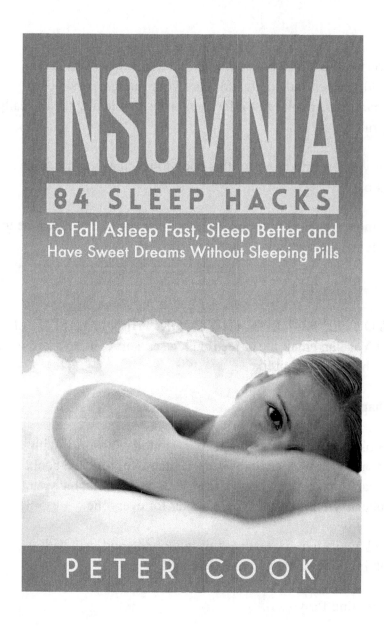

Notes